SCIATICA

CHAIR YOGA

FOR SENIORS OVER 60

A GENTLE AND EFFECTIVE WAY TO RELIEVE SCIATICA SYMPTOMS AT HOME

MARY MORGAN

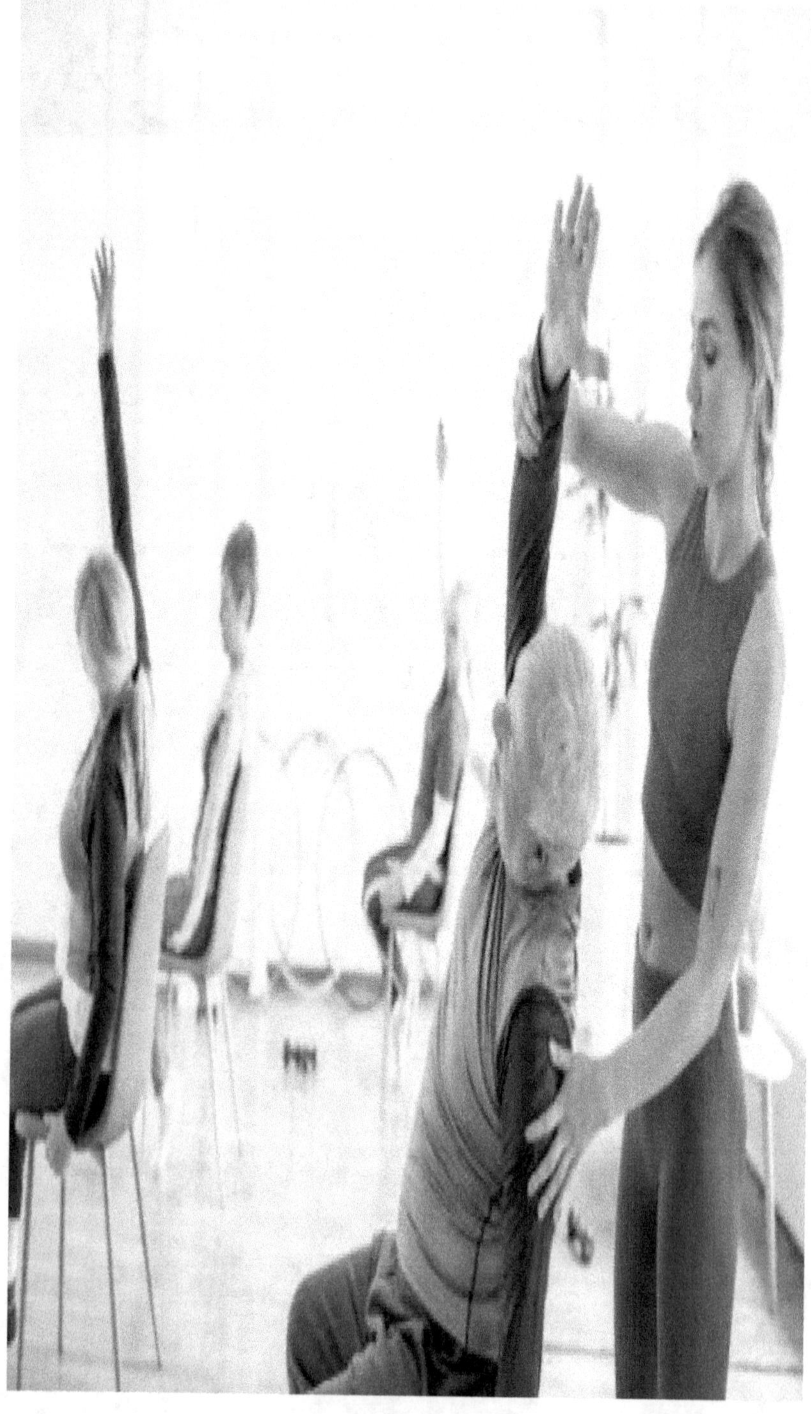

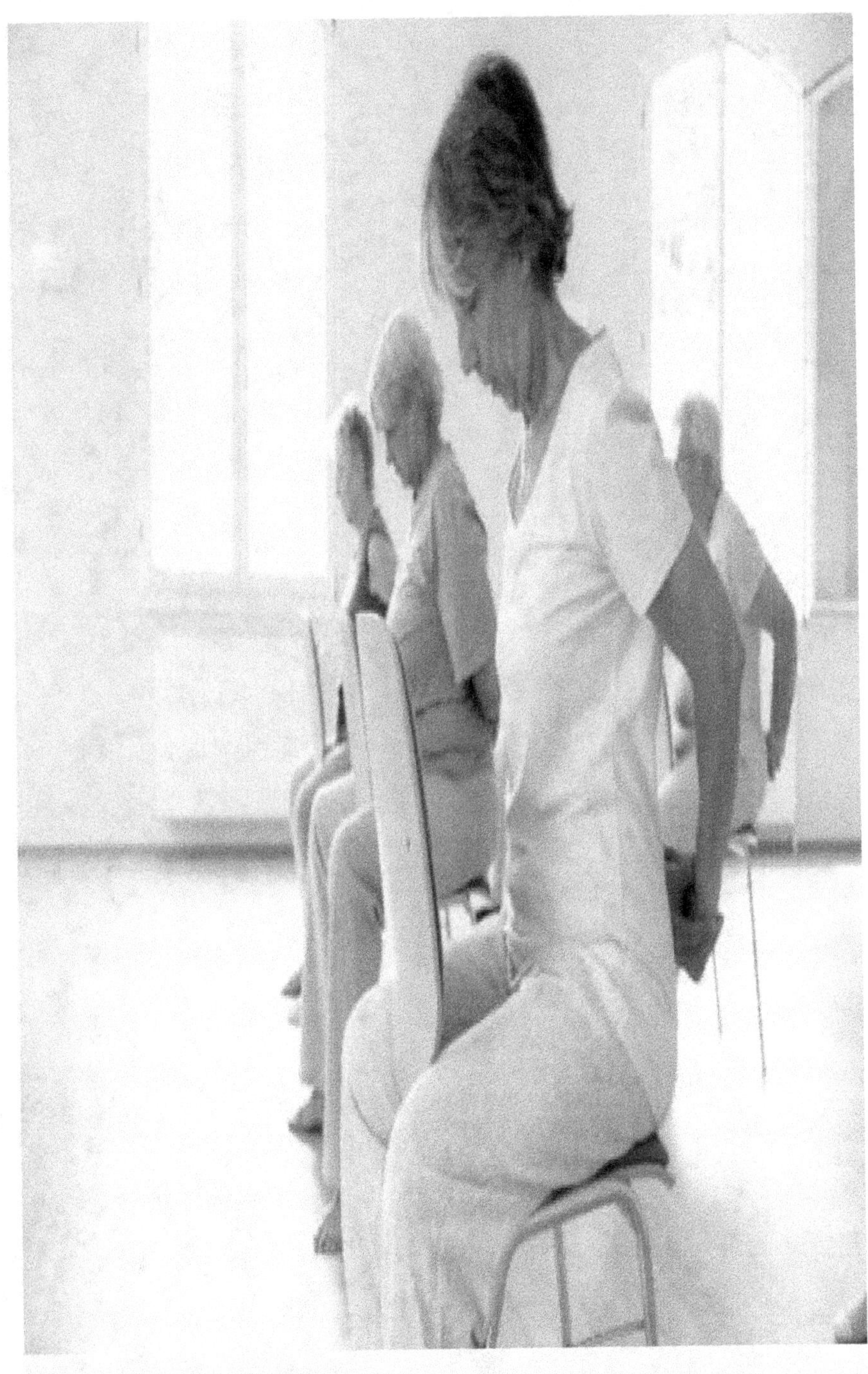

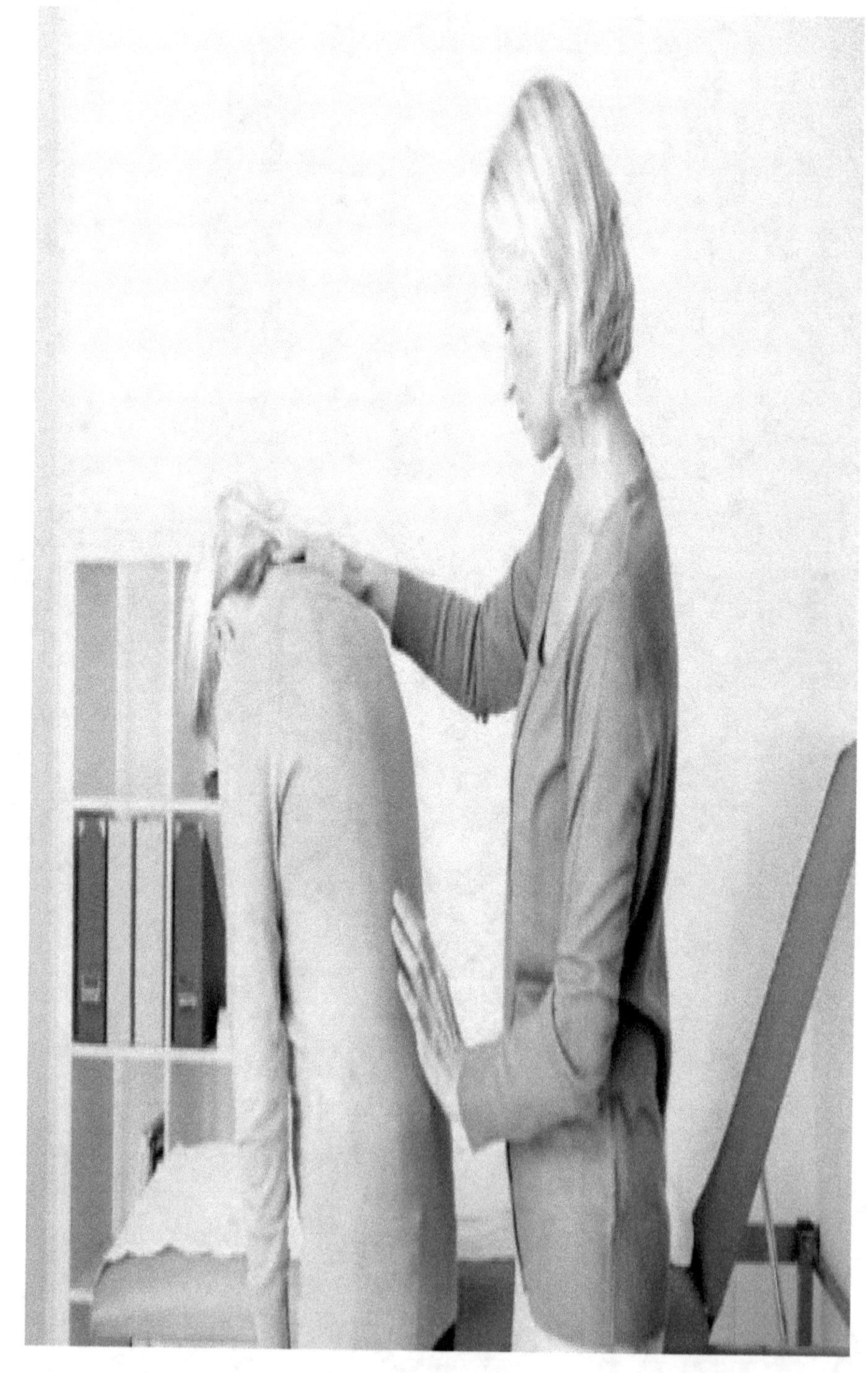

Copyright

CONTENTS

CHAPTER 2: ADVANCED CHAIR YOGA POSES FOR SCIATICA RELIEF

<u>INTRODUCTION:WHAT IS SCIATICA AND WHAT CAUSES IT?</u>

Sciatica is a common condition that affects many people, especially seniors over 60. It is characterized by pain, numbness, tingling, or weakness in the lower back, buttocks, and legs, caused by the compression or irritation of the sciatic nerve. Sciatica can have various causes, such as herniated discs, spinal stenosis, piriformis syndrome, spondylolisthesis, or injury. Sciatica can interfere with your daily activities, mobility, and quality of life, and may require medical attention in some cases.

However, there are also natural and effective ways to relieve sciatica symptoms at home, without the need for surgery, medication, or expensive equipment. One of them is chair yoga, a gentle and accessible form of yoga that can be done by anyone, regardless of age, fitness level, or health condition. Chair yoga involves performing yoga poses and movements while sitting on a chair or using a chair for support. Chair yoga can help you stretch and strengthen your muscles, improve your posture and alignment, increase your blood circulation and oxygen flow, reduce your stress and tension, and enhance your mood and well-being.

In this book, you will learn how to practice chair yoga for sciatica relief, with step-by-step instructions, illustrations, and tips for each pose. You will also find three chair yoga sequences that you can follow along, depending on the time of the day and your energy level and needs. You will also discover some useful tips and precautions to make your chair yoga practice safe and enjoyable. By the end of this book, you will have a better understanding of sciatica and chair yoga, and how they can improve your health and happiness.

This book is suitable for anyone who wants to try chair yoga for sciatica relief, whether you are new to yoga or have some experience. You don't need any special skills or equipment, just a chair and a willingness to learn and have fun. Chair yoga is a wonderful way to take care of yourself, especially if you are a senior over 60 who wants to stay active, flexible, and pain-free.

So, are you ready to start your chair yoga journey? Let's begin!

HOW CAN CHAIR YOGA HELP WITH SCIATICA PAIN AND DISCOMFORT?

Sciatica is a condition that causes pain, numbness, tingling, or weakness in the lower back and legs. It is caused by compression or irritation of the sciatic nerve, which runs from the lower spine to the back of the legs. Sciatica can be triggered by various factors, such as injury, inflammation, herniated disc, spinal stenosis, piriformis syndrome, or pregnancy.

Chair yoga is a form of yoga that can be done while sitting on a chair or using a chair for support. It is suitable for people who have limited mobility, balance issues, or chronic pain.

Chair yoga can help with sciatica pain and discomfort by:

*Stretching and strengthening the muscles and joints in the lower back, hips, and legs, which can reduce pressure on the sciatic nerve and improve blood circulation.

*Improving posture and alignment, which can prevent or correct spinal problems that may contribute to sciatica.

*Relaxing the nervous system and reducing stress, which can ease muscle tension and inflammation that may aggravate sciatica.

*Enhancing mood and well-being, which can boost the body's natural healing abilities and coping skills.

I have been suffering from sciatica for over a year now. It started as a mild ache in my lower back, but soon it became a sharp and shooting pain that radiated down my left leg. I could barely walk, sit, or sleep without feeling the agony of the nerve being pinched. I tried various treatments, such as painkillers, anti-inflammatories, massages, acupuncture, and physiotherapy, but nothing seemed to work. I was losing hope and becoming depressed.

One day, I came across an article online that talked about how chair yoga can help with sciatica pain and discomfort. I was skeptical at first, but I decided to give it a try. I found a local chair yoga class that was suitable for beginners and people with chronic pain. I signed up and went to my first session.

The instructor was very friendly and welcoming. She explained that chair yoga is a form of yoga that can be done while sitting on a chair or using a chair for support. She said that chair yoga can help with sciatica by stretching and strengthening the muscles and joints in the lower back, hips, and legs, improving posture and alignment, relaxing the nervous system and reducing stress, and enhancing mood and well-being. She also assured me that chair yoga is safe and gentle, and that I can modify or skip any poses that are not comfortable for me.

We started with some breathing exercises to calm the mind and body. Then we moved on to some warm-up movements to loosen up the spine and shoulders. Next, we did some chair yoga poses that targeted the areas affected by sciatica, such as seated spinal twist, seated pigeon, and seated forward bend. I was surprised by how much I could stretch and move without feeling any pain or discomfort. I felt a sense of relief and release in my lower back and leg. The instructor guided us through each pose with clear and gentle instructions, and offered some tips and adjustments to make them more effective and accessible. She also encouraged us to listen to our body and breathe deeply throughout the practice.

We ended the session with a relaxation exercise, where we rested our head and chest on a pillow or a blanket on our lap, and closed our eyes. The instructor played some soothing music and spoke some positive affirmations. I felt a wave of peace and gratitude wash over me. I felt like I had just given myself a gift of healing and self-care.

I continued to attend the chair yoga class twice a week for the next two months. I noticed a significant improvement in my sciatica pain and discomfort. I was able to walk, sit, and sleep without any agony. I also felt more flexible, balanced, and confident. I regained my hope and happiness.

Chair yoga has changed my life for the better. It has helped me cope with sciatica pain and discomfort, and also improved my overall health and well-being. I would recommend chair yoga to anyone who is suffering from sciatica or any other chronic pain condition. It is a simple and effective way to heal and restore your body and mind. You don't need any special equipment or experience, just a chair and a willingness to try. Trust me, you won't regret it. SCIATICA Chair yoga for seniors is a miracle!

Chair yoga can be a safe and effective way to help with sciatica pain and discomfort, but it is important to consult with your doctor before starting any new exercise program, especially if you have a medical condition or injury. You should also listen to your body and avoid any poses or movements that cause pain or discomfort. You can modify or skip any poses that are not suitable for you, and use props such as pillows, blankets, or straps to make them more comfortable and accessible. You can also practice chair yoga with a qualified instructor who can guide you and offer personalized adjustments and suggestions. Remember to breathe deeply and enjoy the benefits of chair yoga for your body and mind.

HOW TO USE THIS BOOK AND WHAT YOU WILL NEED

This book is designed to be easy and convenient to use, whether you want to read it from cover to cover or just pick and choose the poses and sequences that suit you best. You can use this book as a guide, a reference, or a source of inspiration for your chair yoga practice. Here are some suggestions on how to

use this book:

Start by reading the introduction, where you will learn more about sciatica and chair yoga, and how they can help you.

Then, move on to chapter 1, where you will find the basic chair yoga poses for sciatica relief. You can try each pose individually, or combine them into your own sequence. Follow the instructions, illustrations, and tips for each pose, and pay attention to your breath, body, and sensations.

Next, proceed to chapter 2, where you will find the advanced chair yoga poses for sciatica relief. These poses are more challenging and require more flexibility and strength. You can practice them after you master the basic poses, or when you feel ready for more variety and intensity. Again, follow the instructions, illustrations, and tips for each pose, and listen to your body and its limits.

After that, explore chapter 3, where you will find three chair yoga sequences for sciatica relief. These sequences are designed to be done at different times of the day, depending on your energy level and needs. You can follow along the sequences as they are, or modify them to suit your preferences and goals. Each sequence has a theme, a duration, and a list of poses, along with a brief description and a reminder of the benefits.

Finally, check out chapter 4, where you will find some useful tips and precautions to make your chair yoga practice safe and enjoyable. You will learn how to breathe properly during chair yoga, how to modify chair yoga poses to suit your needs and abilities, how to avoid common chair yoga mistakes and injuries, how to monitor your progress and pain levels, and when to consult your doctor or a yoga therapist.

As for what you will need, the good news is that chair yoga does not require any special equipment or accessories.

All you need is a chair and some space. Here are some tips on how to choose and prepare your chair and your space:

Choose a chair that is sturdy, stable, and comfortable. Avoid chairs that are too soft, too hard, too high, too low, or too slippery. You can use a dining chair, an office chair, a recliner, or any other chair that works for you.

Make sure your chair has enough space around it, so that you can move your arms and legs freely. You can place your chair near a wall, a table, or another chair for extra support, if needed.

You can also use some props to enhance your chair yoga practice, such as a cushion, a blanket, a towel, a strap, a block, or a pillow. These props can help you adjust your posture, support your joints, deepen your stretch, or add some resistance. You can use items that you already have at home, or buy them online or at a local store.

Wear comfortable clothes that allow you to breathe and move easily. You can wear anything that makes you feel good, such as a T-shirt, a sweater, a pair of pants, or a skirt. You can also wear socks, shoes, or go barefoot, depending on your preference and the temperature.

Find a quiet and relaxing place to do your chair yoga practice, where you can focus on yourself and your breath. You can play some soothing music, light some candles, or use some aromatherapy, if you like. You can also invite a friend, a family member, or a pet to join you, if you want some company and fun.

CHAPTER 1: BASIC CHAIR YOGA POSES FOR SCIATICA RELIEF

In this chapter, you will learn the basic chair yoga poses that can help you relieve sciatica pain and discomfort. These poses are simple and easy to do, and can be done by anyone, regardless of your age, fitness level, or health condition. These poses will help you stretch and strengthen your lower back, buttocks, and legs, where the sciatic nerve runs. They will also help you improve your posture and alignment, which can prevent or reduce the compression or irritation of the sciatic nerve. By practicing these poses regularly, you will feel more relaxed, flexible, and pain-free.

For each pose, you will find the following information:

The name and description of the pose, along with an illustration
The benefits of the pose for sciatica relief
The step-by-step instructions on how to do the pose correctly and safely
The tips and modifications on how to adjust the pose to suit your needs and abilities

The contraindications and precautions on when to avoid or be careful with the pose

Before you start, make sure you have a chair and some space around it. You can also use some props, such as a cushion, a blanket, a towel, a strap, a block, or a pillow, to make your practice more comfortable and effective. You can use items that you already have at home, or buy them online or at a local store.

Remember to breathe deeply and slowly throughout your practice, and pay attention to your body and sensations. Do not force or strain yourself, and respect your limits. If you feel any pain or discomfort, stop or modify the pose. You can also take a break or rest whenever you need to. Listen to your body and its wisdom, and enjoy your practice.

Here are the basic chair yoga poses for sciatica relief:

Seated Mountain Pose

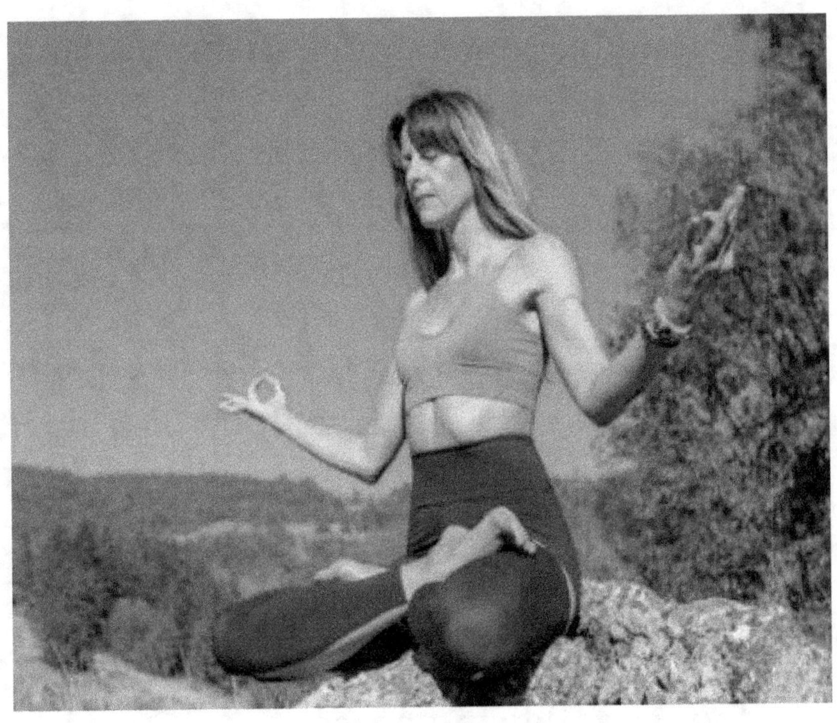

This is a basic sitting posture that helps you establish a good foundation for your chair yoga practice. It helps you align your spine, open your chest, and relax your shoulders and neck. It also helps you become aware of your breath and body.

Benefits

This pose helps you improve your posture and alignment, which can prevent or reduce the compression or irritation of the sciatic nerve. It also helps you calm your mind and nervous system, and prepare yourself for the following poses.

Instructions

Sit on a chair with your feet flat on the floor and your knees bent at 90 degrees. You can place a cushion or a

blanket under your feet or your hips, if needed.

Lengthen your spine and lift your chest. Relax your shoulders and neck. Place your hands on your thighs or on the sides of the chair. Keep your head in line with your spine, and look straight ahead or slightly down.

Breathe deeply and slowly through your nose, and feel your abdomen and chest expand and contract. Focus on your breath and body, and let go of any tension or distraction.

Hold this pose for as long as you like, or for 5 to 10 breaths.

Tips and modifications

You can close your eyes or soften your gaze, if you prefer.

You can place your palms together in front of your chest, or raise your arms overhead, if you want to add some variation and challenge.

You can also sway your torso gently from side to side, or twist your spine slightly to the right and left, if you want to add some movement and stretch.

Contraindications and precautions:

This pose is generally safe and suitable for everyone, but if you have any neck or shoulder issues, be careful not to strain or overextend them.

Seated Forward Bend

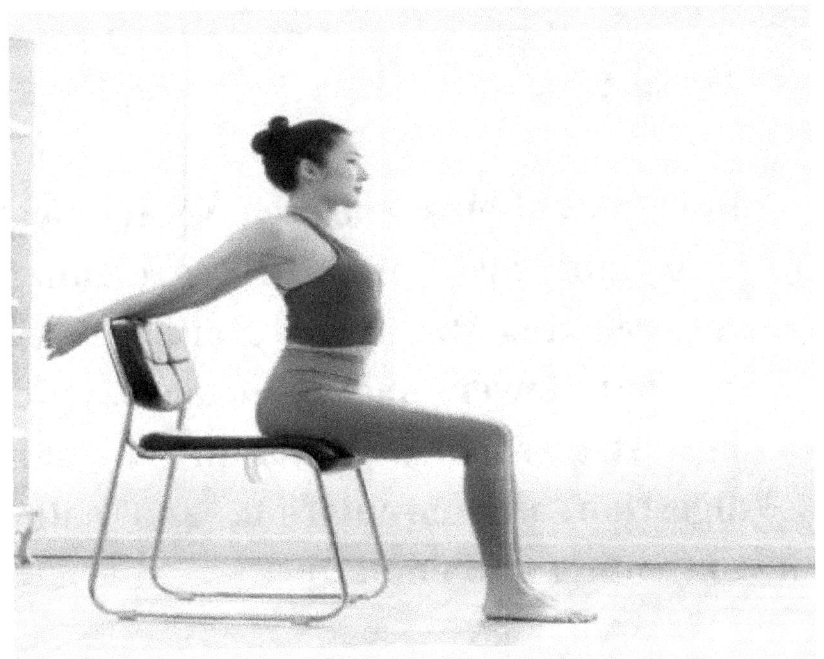

This is a forward folding posture that helps you stretch your lower back, hamstrings, and calves. It also helps you compress your abdomen and massage your internal organs.

Benefits

This pose helps you relieve sciatica pain and discomfort by stretching and relaxing the muscles and nerves in your lower back, buttocks, and legs. It also helps you improve your digestion and circulation, and calm your mind and emotions.

Instructions

Sit on a chair with your feet flat on the floor and your knees bent at 90 degrees. You can place a cushion or a blanket under your feet or your hips, if needed.

Lengthen your spine and lift your chest.

Inhale and raise your arms overhead, or keep them on your thighs or on the sides of the chair

Exhale and hinge from your hips, and fold your torso over your legs. Bring your hands to the floor, to your ankles, to your shins, or to your knees, depending on your flexibility. You can also use a strap, a block, or a pillow to help you reach further, if needed.

- Relax your head, neck, and shoulders, and let them hang loosely. Breathe deeply and slowly through your nose, and feel the stretch in your lower back, hamstrings, and calves. You can also gently rock your head from side to side, or nod your head yes and no, to release any tension or stiffness.

- Hold this pose for as long as you like, or for 5 to 10 breaths.

Tips and modifications

You can bend your knees more or less, depending on your comfort and flexibility.

You can also widen your feet and legs, or cross your legs, if you want to add some variation and intensity.

- You can also wrap your arms around your legs, or interlace your fingers behind your back, if you want to add some movement and stretch.

Contraindications and precautions

This pose is generally safe and suitable for everyone, but if you have any lower back, hip, knee, or hamstring issues, be careful not to overstretch or aggravate them. You can use props or modify the pose to make it more comfortable and safe for you.

If you have any high blood pressure, glaucoma, or heart issues, be careful not to lower your head too much or hold your breath. You can keep your head above your heart, or use props or modify the pose to make it more gentle and safe for you.

Seated Spinal Twist

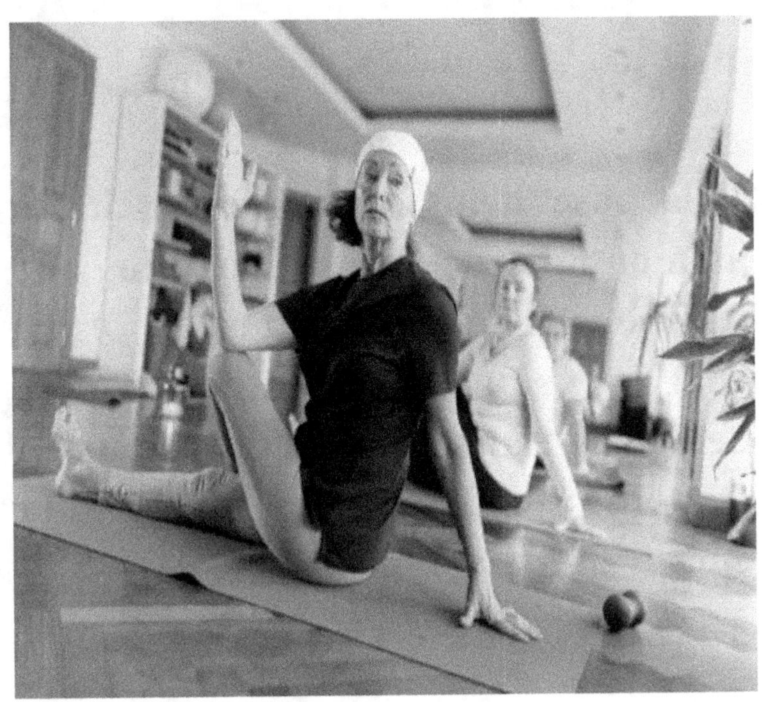

This is a twisting posture that helps you rotate your spine, stretch your back and waist, and stimulate your abdominal organs.

Benefits

This pose helps you relieve sciatica pain and discomfort by loosening and relaxing the muscles and nerves in your lower back and buttocks. It also helps you improve your digestion and detoxification, and balance your energy and emotions.

Instructions

Sit on a chair with your feet flat on the floor and your knees bent at 90 degrees. You can place a cushion or a blanket under your feet or your hips, if needed.

Lengthen your spine and lift your chest. Inhale and raise your arms to shoulder level, or keep them on your thighs or on the sides of the chair.

Exhale and twist your torso to the right, and bring your left hand to the outside of your right knee, and your right hand to the back of the chair or to your right hip. You can also use a strap, a block, or a pillow to help you twist further, if needed.

Keep your hips and legs facing forward, and your shoulders and neck relaxed. Look over your right shoulder, or keep your head in line with your spine, depending on your comfort and flexibility. Breathe deeply and slowly through your nose, and feel the twist in your spine, back, and waist. You can also gently press your left hand against your right knee, or pull your right hand against the back of the chair or your right hip, to deepen the twist.

Hold this pose for as long as you like, or for 5 to 10 breaths.

Inhale and return to the center, and lower your arms. Repeat on the other side.

Tips and modifications

You can bend your knees more or less, depending on your comfort and flexibility.

You can also widen your feet and legs, or cross your legs, if you want to add some variation and intensity.

You can also lift your arms overhead, or interlace your fingers behind your head, if you want to add some movement and stretch.

Contraindications and precautions

This pose is generally safe and suitable for everyone, but if you have any lower back, hip, knee, or spinal issues, be careful not to overtwist or aggravate them. You can use props or modify the pose to make it more comfortable and safe for you.

If you have any high blood pressure, glaucoma, or heart issues, be careful not to twist too much or hold your breath. You can keep your twist gentle and moderate, or use props or modify the pose to make it more gentle and safe for you.

Seated Pigeon Pose

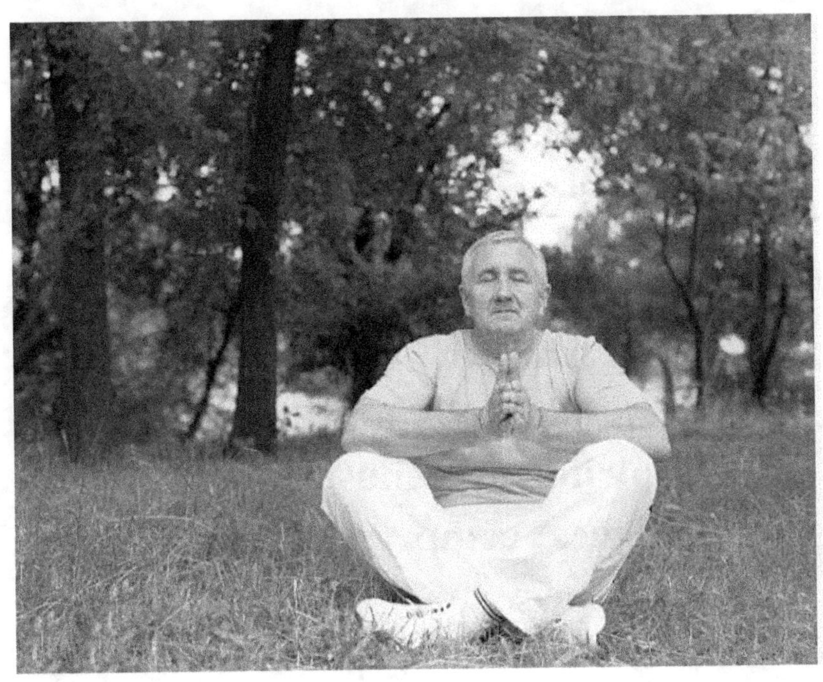

This is a hip opening posture that helps you stretch your outer hips, glutes, and piriformis muscles. It also helps you release any tension or tightness in your pelvic area.

Benefits

This pose helps you relieve sciatica pain and discomfort by stretching and relaxing the muscles and nerves in your buttocks and legs, especially the piriformis muscle, which can sometimes compress or irritate the sciatic nerve. It also helps you improve your hip mobility and stability, and enhance your sexual health and function.

Instructions

Sit on a chair with your feet flat on the floor and your knees bent at 90 degrees. You can place a cushion or a

blanket under your feet or your hips, if needed.

Lengthen your spine and lift your chest. Inhale and lift your right foot off the floor, and place your right ankle on top of your left knee. You can also use a strap, a block, or a pillow to help you lift your foot, if needed.

Flex your right foot and press your right knee down gently. Keep your left foot and leg firmly on the floor. Breathe deeply and slowly through your nose, and feel the stretch in your right outer hip, glute, and piriformis. You can also gently massage your right foot and ankle, or wiggle your toes, to release any tension or stiffness.

If you want to deepen the stretch, exhale and hinge from your hips, and fold your torso over your legs. Bring your hands to the floor, to your ankles, to your shins, or to your knees, depending on your flexibility. You can also use a strap, a block, or a pillow to help you reach further, if needed.

Relax your head, neck, and shoulders, and let them hang loosely. Breathe deeply and slowly through your nose, and feel the stretch in your right outer hip, glute, and piriformis. You can also gently rock your torso from side to side, or twist your spine slightly to the right and left, to add some movement and stretch.

Hold this pose for as long as you like, or for 5 to 10 breaths
Inhale and return to the center, and lower your right foot. Repeat on the other side.

Tips and modifications:

You can bend your knees more or less, depending on your comfort and flexibility.
You can also widen your feet and legs, or cross your legs, if you want to add some variation and intensity.You can also wrap your arms

around your legs, or interlace your fingers behind your back, if you want to add some movement and stretch.

Contraindications and precautions

This pose is generally safe and suitable for everyone, but if you have any lower back, hip, knee, or ankle issues, be careful not to overstretch or aggravate them. You can use props or modify the pose to make it more comfortable and safe for you.

If you have any high blood pressure, glaucoma, or heart issues, be careful not to lower your head too much or hold your breath. You can keep your head above your heart, or use props or modify the pose to make it more gentle and safe for you.

Seated Cat-Cow Stretch

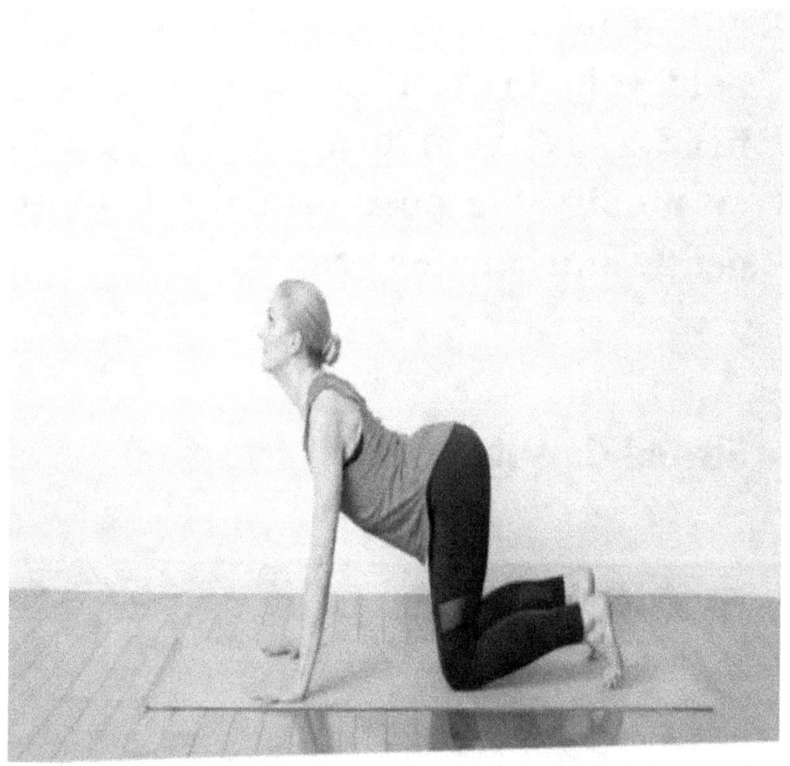

This is a spinal movement that helps you flex and extend your spine, stretch your back and chest, and stimulate your abdominal organs.

Benefits

This pose helps you relieve sciatica pain and discomfort by loosening and relaxing the muscles and nerves in your lower back and buttocks. It also helps you improve your spinal mobility and flexibility, and balance your energy and emotions.

Instructions

Sit on a chair with your feet flat on the floor and your knees bent at 90 degrees. You can place a cushion or a blanket under your feet or your hips, if needed.

Lengthen your spine and lift your chest. Place your hands on your thighs or on the sides of the chair. Keep your head in line with your spine, and look straight ahead or slightly down.

Inhale and arch your back, and lift your chest and chin. This is the cow pose. Breathe deeply and slowly through your nose, and feel the stretch in your back and chest. You can also gently squeeze your shoulder blades together, or lift your arms overhead, to deepen the stretch. Exhale and round your back, and tuck your chest and chin. This is the cat pose. Breathe deeply and slowly through your nose, and feel the stretch in your back and chest. You can also gently press your hands against your thighs, or bring your arms in front of you, to deepen the stretch.

Repeat this movement for as long as you like, or for 5 to 10 times.

Tips and modifications:

You can bend your knees more or less, depending on your comfort and flexibility.

You can also widen your feet and legs, or cross your legs, if you want to add some variation and intensity.
You can also move your head and neck along with your spine, or keep

them still, depending on your comfort and flexibility.

Contraindications and precautions

This pose is generally safe and suitable for everyone, but if you have any lower back, neck, or spinal issues, be careful not to overarch or overround your spine. You can use props or modify the pose to make it more comfortable and safe for you.

If you have any high blood pressure, glaucoma, or heart issues, be careful not to lift or lower your head too much or hold your breath. You can keep your head in line with your spine, or use props or modify the pose to make it more gentle and safe for you.

Seated Side Stretch

This is a lateral bending posture that helps you stretch your sides, waist, and ribs. It also helps you open your lungs and breathe more deeply.

Benefits

This pose helps you relieve sciatica pain and discomfort by stretching and relaxing the muscles and nerves in your lower back and buttocks. It also helps you improve your posture and alignment, and enhance your oxygen intake and energy level.

Instructions

Sit on a chair with your feet flat on the floor and your knees bent at 90 degrees. You can place a cushion or a blanket under your feet or your hips, if needed.

Lengthen your spine and lift your chest. Inhale and raise your arms overhead, or keep them on your thighs or on the sides of the chair.

Exhale and bend your torso to the right, and bring your right hand to the right side of the chair or to your right hip, and your left hand to the right side of your head or to your left ear. You can also use a strap, a block, or a pillow to help you bend further, if needed.

CHAPTER 2: Advanced Chair Yoga Poses for Sciatica Relief

In this chapter, you will learn the advanced chair yoga poses that can help you relieve sciatica pain and discomfort. These poses are more challenging and require more flexibility and strength than the basic poses. You can practice them after you master the basic poses, or when you feel ready for more variety and intensity. These poses will help you stretch and strengthen your lower back, buttocks, and legs, where the sciatic nerve runs. They will also help you improve your posture and alignment, which can prevent or reduce the compression or irritation of the sciatic nerve. By practicing these poses regularly, you will feel more relaxed, flexible, and pain-free.

For each pose, you will find the following information:

The name and description of the pose, along with an illustration

The benefits of the pose for sciatica relief
The step-by-step instructions on how to do the pose correctly and safely

The tips and modifications on how to adjust the pose to suit your needs and abilities

The contraindications and precautions on when to avoid or be careful with the pose

Before you start, make sure you have a chair and some space around it. You can also use some props, such as a cushion, a blanket, a towel, a strap, a block, or a pillow, to make your practice more comfortable and effective. You can use items that you already have at home, or buy them online or at a local store.

Remember to breathe deeply and slowly throughout your practice, and pay attention to your body and sensations. Do not force or strain yourself, and respect your limits. If you feel any pain or discomfort, stop or modify the pose. You can also take a break or rest whenever you need to. Listen to your body and its wisdom, and enjoy your practice.

Here are the advanced chair yoga poses for sciatica relief:

Seated Eagle Pose (Garudasana)

This is a balancing and twisting posture that helps you cross and wrap your limbs around each other. It helps you stretch your outer hips, glutes, and piriformis muscles, as well as your upper back, shoulders, and arms.

Benefits

This pose helps you relieve sciatica pain and discomfort by stretching and relaxing the muscles and nerves in your buttocks and legs, especially the piriformis muscle, which can sometimes compress or irritate the sciatic nerve. It also helps you improve your balance, coordination, and concentration, and release any stress or tension.

Instructions:

Sit on a chair with your feet flat on the floor and your knees bent at 90 degrees. You can place a cushion or a blanket under your feet or your hips, if needed.

Lengthen your spine and lift your chest. Inhale and raise your arms to shoulder level, or keep them on your thighs or on the sides of the chair.

Exhale and cross your right arm over your left arm, and wrap your arms around each other. Bring your palms together, or touch the backs of your hands, depending on your flexibility. You can also use a strap, a block, or a pillow to help you wrap your arms, if needed.

Keep your elbows at shoulder level, and your shoulders and neck relaxed. Breathe deeply and slowly through your nose, and feel the stretch in your upper back, shoulders, and arms. You can also gently press your palms together, or pull your hands away from each other, to deepen the stretch.

If you want to add the leg variation, exhale and cross your right leg over your left leg, and wrap your legs around each other. Hook your right foot behind your left calf, or touch the top of your right foot to the floor, depending on your flexibility. You can also use a strap, a block, or a pillow to help you wrap your legs, if needed.

Keep your hips and pelvis facing forward, and your spine and chest lifted. Breathe deeply and slowly through your nose, and feel the stretch in your outer hips, glutes, and piriformis. You can also gently press your right knee down, or pull your left knee up, to deepen the stretch.

Hold this pose for as long as you like, or for 5 to 10 breaths.
 Inhale and unwind your arms and legs. Repeat on the other side.

Tips and modifications:

You can bend your knees more or less, depending on your comfort and flexibility.

You can also widen your feet and legs, or cross your legs, if you want to add some variation and intensity.

You can also twist your torso slightly to the right and left, or tilt your head slightly to the right and left, if you want to add some movement and stretch.

Contraindications and precautions

This pose is generally safe and suitable for everyone, but if you have any lower back, hip, knee, ankle, shoulder, or wrist issues, be careful not to overcross or overwrap your limbs. You can use props or modify the pose to make it more comfortable and safe for you.

If you have any high blood pressure, glaucoma, or heart issues, be careful not to hold your breath or tighten your chest. You can keep your breath smooth and steady, or use props or modify the pose to make it more gentle and safe for you.

Seated Half Moon Pose (Ardha Chandrasana)

This is a lateral bending posture that helps you stretch your sides, waist, and ribs. It also helps you open your lungs and breathe more deeply.

Benefits

This pose helps you relieve sciatica pain and discomfort by stretching and relaxing the muscles and nerves in your lower back and buttocks. It also helps you improve your posture and alignment, and enhance your oxygen intake and energy level.

Instructions:

Sit on a chair with your feet flat on the floor and your knees bent at 90 degrees. You can place a cushion or a blanket under your feet or your hips, if needed.

Lengthen your spine and lift your chest. Inhale and raise your arms overhead, or keep them on your thighs or on the sides of the chair.

Exhale and bend your torso to the right, and bring your right hand to the right side of the chair or to your right hip, and your left hand to the right side of your head or to your left ear. You can also use a strap, a block, or a pillow to help you bend further, if needed.

Keep your hips and legs facing forward, and your shoulders and neck relaxed. Look up at your left hand, or keep your head in line with your spine, depending on your comfort and flexibility. Breathe deeply and slowly through your nose, and feel the stretch in your left side, waist, and ribs. You can also gently pull your left hand away from your head, or press your right hand against the chair or your hip, to deepen the stretch.

Hold this pose for as long as you like, or for 5 to 10 breaths.

Inhale and return to the center, and raise your arms. Repeat on the other side.

Tips and modifications:

You can bend your knees more or less, depending on your comfort and flexibility.

You can also widen your feet and legs, or cross your legs, if you want to add some variation and intensity.

You can also twist your torso slightly to the right and left, or nod your head yes and no, if you want to add some movement and stretch.

Contraindications and precautions

This pose is generally safe and suitable for everyone, but if you have any lower back, hip, knee, or spinal issues, be careful not to overbend or aggravate them. You can use props or modify the pose to make it more comfortable and safe for you.

If you have any high blood pressure, glaucoma, or heart issues, be careful not to lift or lower your head too much or hold your breath. You can keep your head in line with your spine, or use props or modify the pose to make it more gentle and safe for you.

Seated Warrior I and II (Virabhadrasana I and II)

These are standing postures that help you stretch your legs, hips, and groin, and strengthen your core, back, and arms. They also help you open your chest and shoulders, and improve your balance and stability.

Benefits

These poses help you relieve sciatica pain and discomfort by stretching and relaxing the muscles and nerves in your lower back, buttocks, and legs. They also help you improve your posture and alignment, and enhance your confidence and courage.

Instructions

Sit on a chair with your feet flat on the floor and your knees bent at 90 degrees. You can place a cushion or a blanket under your feet or your hips, if needed.

Lengthen your spine and lift your chest. Inhale and raise your arms overhead, or keep them on your thighs or on the sides of the chair.

Exhale and slide your right foot back, and place your right heel on the floor, at a 45-degree angle. Keep your left foot and leg firmly on the floor, and your left knee bent at 90 degrees.

This is the warrior I pose. Breathe deeply and slowly through your nose, and feel the stretch in your right leg, hip, and groin. You can also gently press your right heel against the floor, or pull your left knee over your left ankle, to deepen the stretch.

If you want to add the arm variation, inhale and raise your arms overhead, and bring your palms together, or keep them shoulder-width apart, depending on your flexibility. You can also use a strap, a block, or a pillow to help you raise your arms, if needed.

Keep your hips and pelvis facing forward, and your shoulders and neck relaxed. Look up at your hands, or keep your head in line with your spine, depending on your comfort and flexibility. Breathe deeply and slowly through your nose, and feel the stretch in your chest and shoulders. You can also gently press your palms together, or pull your hands away from each other, to deepen the stretch.

Hold this pose for as long as you like, or for 5 to 10 breaths.

To transition to the warrior II pose, exhale and lower your arms to shoulder level, and turn your torso to the right. Keep your right foot and leg as they are, and your left foot and leg firmly on the floor, and your left knee bent at 90 degrees.

 Keep your hips and pelvis facing the right, and your shoulders and neck relaxed. Look over your left hand, or keep your head in line with your spine, depending on your comfort and flexibility. Breathe deeply and slowly through your nose, and feel the stretch in your legs, hips, and groin. You can also gently press your right heel against the floor, or pull your left knee over your left ankle, to deepen the stretch.

Hold this pose for as long as you like, or for 5 to 10 breaths.

Inhale and return to the center, and raise your arms. Repeat on the other side.

Tips and modifications

You can bend your knees more or less, depending on your comfort and flexibility.

You can also widen your feet and legs, or cross your legs, if you want to add some variation and intensity.

You can also twist your torso slightly to the right and left, or tilt your head slightly to the right and left, if you want to add some movement and stretch.

Contraindications and precautions

These poses are generally safe and suitable for everyone, but if you have any lower back, hip, knee, or ankle issues, be careful not to overstretch or aggravate them. You can use props or modify the pose to make it more comfortable and safe for you.

If you have any high blood pressure, glaucoma, or heart issues, be careful not to lift or lower your head too much or hold your breath. You can keep your head in line with your spine, or use props or modify the pose to make it more gentle and safe for you.

CHAPTER 3: Chair Yoga Sequences for Sciatica Relief

In this section, you will find three chair yoga sequences that you can follow along, depending on the time of the day and your energy level and needs. These sequences are composed of the basic and advanced chair yoga poses that you have learned in the previous chapters, as well as some additional poses that can complement and enhance your practice. These sequences will help you relieve sciatica pain and discomfort, as well as improve your overall health and well-being.

For each sequence, you will find the following information:

The name and theme of the sequence, along with an illustration

- The duration and difficulty level of the sequence

- The list of poses and movements that are included in the sequence, along with a brief description and a reminder of the benefits

- The step-by-step instructions on how to do the sequence correctly and safely

- The tips and modifications on how to adjust the sequence to suit your needs and abilities
-    The contraindications and precautions on when to avoid or be careful with the sequence

Before you start, make sure you have a chair and some space around it. You can also use some props, such as a cushion, a blanket, a towel, a strap, a block, or a pillow, to make your practice more comfortable and effective. You can use items that you already have at home, or buy them online or at a local store.

Remember to breathe deeply and slowly throughout your practice, and pay attention to your body and sensations. Do not force or strain yourself, and respect your limits. If you feel any pain or discomfort, stop or modify the pose or the sequence. You can also take a break or rest whenever you need to. Listen to your body and its wisdom, and enjoy your practice.

Here are the chair yoga sequences for sciatica relief:

Morning Chair Yoga Sequence for Sciatica Relief

This is a sequence that you can do in the morning, or anytime you want to start your day with some energy and positivity. It helps you wake up your body and mind, and prepare yourself for the day ahead. It also helps you relieve sciatica pain and discomfort, and improve your mood and motivation.

Duration and difficulty: This sequence takes about 15 to 20 minutes, and is suitable for beginners and intermediate practitioners.

Poses and movements

This sequence includes the following poses and movements:

Seated Mountain Pose:

This is a basic sitting posture that helps you establish a good foundation for your chair yoga practice. It helps you align your spine, open your chest, and relax your shoulders and neck. It also helps you become aware of your breath and body. (See Chapter 1 for more details)

Seated Cat-Cow Stretch

This is a spinal movement that helps you flex and extend your spine, stretch your back and chest, and stimulate your abdominal organs. It also helps you loosen and relax the muscles and nerves in your lower back and buttocks. (See Chapter 1 for more details)

Seated Side Stretch

This is a lateral bending posture that helps you stretch your sides, waist, and ribs. It also helps you open your lungs and breathe more deeply. It also helps you stretch and relax the muscles and nerves in your lower back and buttocks. (See Chapter 1 for more details)

Seated Eagle Pose

This is a balancing and twisting posture that helps you cross and wrap your limbs around each other. It helps you stretch your outer hips, glutes, and piriformis muscles, as well as your upper back, shoulders, and arms. It also helps you improve your balance, coordination, and concentration, and release any stress or tension. (See Chapter 2 for more details)

Seated Warrior I and II

These are standing postures that help you stretch your legs, hips, and groin, and strengthen your core, back, and arms. They also help you open your chest and shoulders, and improve your balance and stability. They also help you stretch and relax the muscles and nerves in your lower back, buttocks, and legs. (See Chapter 2 for more details)

Seated Sun Salutation

This is a series of poses and movements that help you warm up your body and mind, and synchronize your breath and movement. It helps you stretch and strengthen your whole body, and improve your circulation and oxygen flow. It also helps you relieve sciatica pain and discomfort, and enhance your energy and vitality. (See below for more details)

Instructions

Sit on a chair with your feet flat on the floor and your knees bent at 90 degrees. You can place a cushion or a blanket under your feet or your hips, if needed.

Lengthen your spine and lift your chest. Place your hands on your thighs or on the sides of the chair. Keep your head in line with your spine, and look straight ahead or slightly down.

Breathe deeply and slowly through your nose, and feel your abdomen and chest expand and contract. Focus on your breath and body, and let go of any tension or distraction.

Begin with the Seated Mountain Pose, and hold it for 5 to 10 breaths. Then, move on to the Seated Cat-Cow Stretch, and repeat it for 5 to 10 times. Next, proceed to the Seated Side Stretch, and hold it for 5 to 10 breaths on each side. After that, explore the Seated Eagle Pose, and hold it for 5 to 10 breaths on each side. Then, transition to the Seated Warrior I and II, and hold them for 5 to 10 breaths on each side. Finally, end with the Seated Sun Salutation, and repeat it for 3 to 5 times.

Follow the instructions, illustrations, and tips for each pose and movement, as described in the previous chapters, or see below for the Seated Sun Salutation. Pay attention to your breath, body, and sensations. Do not force or strain yourself, and respect your limits. If you feel any pain or discomfort, stop or modify the pose or the sequence. You can also take a break or rest whenever you need to.

To do the Seated Sun Salutation, follow these steps:

Inhale and raise your arms overhead, and bring your palms together. Look up at your hands, or keep your head in line with your spine. This is the Seated Mountain Pose with Prayer Hands.

Exhale and hinge from your hips, and fold your torso over your legs. Bring your hands to the floor, to your ankles, to your shins, or to your knees. Relax your head, neck, and shoulders. This is the Seated Forward Bend.

Inhale and lift your torso halfway up, and place your hands on your shins or on the sides of the chair. Lengthen your spine and lift your chest. Look straight ahead or slightly down. This is the Seated Halfway Lift.

Exhale and fold your torso over your legs again. Bring your hands to the floor, to your ankles, to your shins, or to your knees. Relax your head, neck, and shoulders. This is the Seated Forward Bend.

Inhale and raise your torso and arms up, and bring your palms together. Look up at your hands, or keep your head in line with your spine. This is the Seated Mountain Pose with Prayer Hands.

Exhale and lower your arms to shoulder level, and turn your torso to the right. Bring your left hand to the outside of your right knee, and your right hand to the back of the chair or to your right hip. Look over your right shoulder, or keep your head in line with your spine. This is the Seated Spinal Twist to the right. (See Chapter 1 for more details)

Inhale and return to the center, and raise your arms to shoulder level. This is the Seated Mountain Pose with Arms Out.

Exhale and turn your torso to the left. Bring your right hand to the outside of your left knee, and your left hand to the back of the chair or to your left hip. Look over your left shoulder, or keep your head in line with your spine. This is the Seated Spinal Twist to the left. (See Chapter 1 for more details)

Inhale and return to the center, and lower your arms. This is the Seated Mountain Pose.

Repeat the whole sequence from the beginning, or move on to the next pose or sequence.

Tips and modifications

You can adjust the duration and difficulty of the sequence, depending on your time, energy, and ability. You can do more or less repetitions, or hold the poses for longer or shorter periods of time. You can also skip or add some poses or movements, depending on your preference and goals.

You can also use some props, such as a cushion, a blanket, a towel, a strap, a block, or a pillow, to make your practice more comfortable and effective. You can use items that you already have at home, or buy them online or at a local store.

You can also play some uplifting music, light some candles, or use some aromatherapy, if you like. You can also invite a friend, a family member, or a pet to join you, if you want some company and fun.

Contraindications and precautions:

This sequence is generally safe and suitable for everyone, but if you have any medical or health issues, consult your

doctor or a yoga therapist before doing this sequence, or any other chair yoga practice. You can also ask them for advice on how to modify the sequence to suit your specific needs and conditions.

If you have any lower back, hip, knee, ankle, shoulder, wrist, neck, or spinal issues, be careful not to overstretch or aggravate them. You can use props or modify the pose or the sequence to make it more comfortable and safe for you.

If you have any high blood pressure, glaucoma, or heart issues, be careful not to lift or lower your head too much or hold your breath. You can keep your head in line with your spine, or use props or modify the pose or the sequence to make it more gentle and safe for you.

Afternoon Chair Yoga Sequence for Sciatica Relief

This is a sequence that you can do in the afternoon, or anytime you want to take a break from your daily activities and refresh yourself. It helps you relax your body and mind, and release any tension or fatigue. It also helps you relieve sciatica pain and discomfort, and improve your mood and focus.

Duration and difficulty

This sequence takes about 15 to 20 minutes, and is suitable for beginners and intermediate practitioners.

Poses and movements

This sequence includes the following poses and movements:

- Seated Mountain Pose: This is a basic sitting posture that helps you establish a good foundation for your chair yoga practice. It helps you align your spine, open your chest, and relax your shoulders and neck. It also helps you become aware of your breath and body. (See Chapter 1 for more details)

Seated Neck Stretch

This is a simple movement that helps you stretch your neck and shoulders, and release any stiffness or soreness. It also helps you relax your mind and nervous system, and ease any headache or stress. (See below for more details)

Seated Shoulder Roll

This is a simple movement that helps you rotate your shoulders, and loosen and lubricate your shoulder joints. It also helps you open your chest and shoulders, and improve your posture and breathing. (See below for more details)

Seated Pigeon Pose

This is a hip opening posture that helps you stretch your outer hips, glutes, and piriformis muscles. It also helps you release any tension or tightness in your pelvic area. It also helps you stretch and relax the muscles and nerves in your buttocks and legs, especially the piriformis muscle, which can sometimes compress or irritate the sciatic nerve. (See Chapter 1 for more details)

Seated Half Moon Pose:

This is a lateral bending posture that helps you stretch your sides, waist, and ribs. It also helps you open your lungs and breathe more deeply. It also helps you stretch and relax the muscles and nerves in your lower back and buttocks. (See Chapter 2 for more details)

Seated Extended Triangle Pose: This is a standing posture that helps you stretch your legs, hips, and groin, and strengthen your core, back, and arms. It also helps you open your chest and shoulders, and improve your balance and stability. It also helps you stretch and relax the muscles and nerves in your lower back, buttocks, and legs. (See Chapter 2 for more details)

Seated Bridge Pose: This is a backbending posture that helps you lift your hips and chest, and stretch your front body. It also helps you strengthen your core, back, and legs, and stimulate your thyroid and adrenal glands. It also helps you stretch and relax the muscles and nerves in your lower back and buttocks. (See Chapter 2 for more details)

- Seated Fish Pose: This is a backbending posture that helps you arch your back and open your chest and throat. It also helps you stretch your neck and shoulders, and stimulate your thyroid and parathyroid glands. It also helps you stretch and relax the muscles and nerves in your lower back and buttocks. (See Chapter 2 for more details)

Instructions

Sit on a chair with your feet flat on the floor and your knees bent at 90 degrees. You can place a cushion or a blanket under your feet or your hips, if needed.

- Lengthen your spine and lift your chest. Place your hands on your thighs or on the sides of the chair. Keep your head in line with your spine, and look straight ahead or slightly down.

- Breathe deeply and slowly through your nose, and feel your abdomen and chest expand and contract. Focus on your breath and body, and let go of any tension or distraction.

- Begin with the Seated Mountain Pose, and hold it for 5 to 10 breaths. Then, move on to the Seated Neck Stretch, and repeat it for 5 to 10 times on each side. Next, proceed to the Seated Shoulder Roll, and repeat it for 5 to 10 times in each direction. After that, explore the Seated Pigeon Pose, and hold it for 5 to 10 breaths on each side. Then, transition to the Seated Half Moon Pose, and hold it for 5 to 10 breaths on each side. Next, proceed to the Seated Extended Triangle Pose, and hold it for 5 to 10 breaths on each side. After that, explore the Seated Bridge Pose, and hold it for 5 to 10 breaths. Finally, end with the Seated Fish Pose, and hold it for 5 to 10 breaths.

Follow the instructions, illustrations, and tips for each pose and movement, as described in the previous chapters, or see below for the Seated Neck Stretch and the Seated Shoulder Roll. Pay attention to your breath, body, and sensations. Do not force or strain yourself, and respect your limits. If you feel any pain or discomfort, stop or modify the pose or the sequence. You can also take a break or rest whenever you need to.

To do the Seated Neck Stretch, follow these steps:

- Inhale and lengthen your spine and lift your chest. Place your hands on your thighs or on the sides of the chair. Keep your head in line with your spine, and look straight ahead or slightly down. This is the Seated Mountain Pose.

- Exhale and lower your right ear to your right shoulder, and bring your right hand to the left side of your head or to your left ear. You can also use a strap, a block, or a pillow to help you lower your ear, if needed.

- Keep your left shoulder down and relaxed, and your left hand on your thigh or on the side of the chair. Breathe deeply and slowly through your nose, and feel the stretch in your left neck and shoulder. You can also gently pull your right ear closer to your right shoulder, or press your left hand against the chair or your thigh, to deepen the stretch.

Hold this pose for as long as you like, or for 5 to 10 breaths.

Inhale and return to the center, and lower your right hand. Repeat on the other side.

To do the Seated Shoulder Roll, follow these steps:
- Inhale and lengthen your spine and lift your chest. Place your hands on your thighs or on the sides of the chair. Keep your head in line with your spine, and look straight ahead or slightly down. This is the Seated Mountain Pose.

Exhale and roll your shoulders up, back, down, and forward, in a circular motion. Breathe deeply and slowly through your nose, and feel the movement and lubrication in your shoulder joints. You can also gently squeeze your shoulder blades together, or lift your arms overhead, to add some variation and stretch.

Repeat this movement for as long as you like, or for 5 to 10 times in one direction. Then, reverse the direction, and repeat for 5 to 10 times in the opposite direction.

Tips and modifications

You can adjust the duration and difficulty of the sequence, depending on your time, energy, and ability. You can do more or less repetitions, or hold the poses for longer or shorter periods of time. You can also skip or add some poses or movements, depending on your preference and goals.

- You can also use some props, such as a cushion, a blanket, a towel, a strap, a block, or a pillow, to make your practice more comfortable and effective. You can use items that you already have at home, or buy them online or at a local store.

- You can also play some relaxing music, light some candles, or use some aromatherapy, if you like. You can also invite a friend, a family member, or a pet to join you, if you want some company and fun.

Contraindications and precautions

This sequence is generally safe and suitable for everyone, but if you have any medical or health issues, consult your doctor or a yoga therapist before doing this sequence, or any other chair yoga practice. You can also ask them for advice on how to modify the sequence to suit your

You can also ask them for advice on how to modify the sequence to suit your specific needs and conditions.

If you have any lower back, hip, knee, ankle, shoulder, wrist, neck, or spinal issues, be careful not to overstretch or aggravate them. You can use props or modify the pose or the sequence to make it more comfortable and safe for you.

If you have any high blood pressure, glaucoma, or heart issues, be careful not to lift or lower your head too much or hold your breath. You can keep your head in line with your spine, or use props or modify the pose or the sequence to make it more gentle and safe for you.

Here is a possible section on "Evening Chair Yoga Sequence for Sciatica Relief" for a book on "Sciatica chair yoga for seniors over 60: a gentle and effective way to relieve sciatica symptoms at home":

Evening Chair Yoga Sequence for Sciatica Relief

- This is a sequence that you can do in the evening, or anytime you want to wind down your day and prepare yourself for a good night's sleep. It helps you relax your body and mind, and release any stress or anxiety. It also helps you relieve sciatica pain and discomfort, and improve your sleep quality and duration.

- Duration and difficulty: This sequence takes about 15 to 20 minutes, and is suitable for beginners and intermediate practitioners.

Poses and movements

This sequence includes the following poses and movements:

- Seated Mountain Pose: This is a basic sitting posture that helps you establish a good foundation for your chair yoga practice. It helps you align your spine, open your chest, and relax your shoulders and neck. It also helps you become aware of your breath and body. (See Chapter 1 for more details)

- Seated Forward Bend: This is a forward folding posture that helps you stretch your lower back, hamstrings, and calves. It also helps you compress your abdomen and massage your internal organs. It also helps you stretch and relax the muscles and nerves in your lower back, buttocks, and legs. (See Chapter 1 for more details)

Seated Spinal Twist

This is a twisting posture that helps you rotate your spine, stretch your back and waist, and stimulate your abdominal organs. It also helps you loosen and relax the muscles and nerves in your lower back and buttocks. (See Chapter 1 for more details)

Seated Pigeon Pose

This is a hip opening posture that helps you stretch your outer hips, glutes, and piriformis muscles. It also helps you release any tension or tightness in your pelvic area. It also helps you stretch and relax the muscles and nerves in your buttocks and legs, especially the piriformis muscle, which can sometimes compress or irritate the sciatic nerve. (See Chapter 1 for more details)

Seated Bridge Pose

This is a backbending posture that helps you lift your hips and chest, and stretch your front body. It also helps you strengthen your core, back, and legs, and stimulate your thyroid and adrenal glands. It also helps you stretch and relax the muscles and nerves in your lower back and buttocks. (See Chapter 2 for more details)

Seated Fish Pose

This is a backbending posture that helps you arch your back and open your chest and throat. It also helps you stretch your neck and shoulders, and stimulate your thyroid and parathyroid glands. It also helps you stretch and relax the muscles and nerves in your lower back and buttocks. (See Chapter 2 for more details)

Seated Meditation

This is a simple practice that helps you calm your mind and body, and cultivate awareness and mindfulness. It also helps you relax your nervous system, and ease any pain or discomfort. (See below for more details)

Instructions

Sit on a chair with your feet flat on the floor and your knees bent at 90 degrees. You can place a cushion or a blanket under your feet or your hips, if needed.

Lengthen your spine and lift your chest. Place your hands on your thighs or on the sides of the chair. Keep your head in line with your spine, and look straight ahead or slightly down.
Breathe deeply and slowly through your nose, and feel your abdomen and chest expand and contract. Focus on your breath and body, and let go of any tension or distraction.

Begin with the Seated Mountain Pose, and hold it for 5 to 10 breaths. Then, move on to the Seated Forward Bend, and hold it for 5 to 10 breaths. Next, proceed to the Seated Spinal Twist, and hold it for 5 to 10 breaths on each side. After that, explore the Seated Pigeon Pose, and hold it for 5 to 10 breaths on each side. Then, transition to the Seated Bridge Pose, and hold it for 5 to 10 breaths. Next, proceed to the Seated Fish Pose, and hold it for 5 to 10 breaths. Finally, end with the Seated Meditation, and hold it for as long as you like, or for 5 to 10 minutes.

Follow the instructions, illustrations, and tips for each pose and movement, as described in the previous chapters, or see below for the Seated Meditation. Pay attention to your breath, body, and sensations. Do not force or strain yourself, and respect your limits. If you feel any pain or discomfort, stop or modify the pose or the sequence. You can also take a break or rest whenever you need to.

To do the Seated Meditation, follow these steps:

Inhale and lengthen your spine and lift your chest. Place your hands on your thighs or on the sides of the chair. Keep your head in line with your spine, and look straight ahead or slightly down. This is the Seated Mountain Pose.

Exhale and close your eyes or soften your gaze, and relax your face and jaw. Breathe deeply and slowly through your nose, and feel your abdomen and chest expand and contract. Focus on your breath and body, and let go of any thoughts or emotions.

Stay in this state of awareness and mindfulness, and observe your breath and body, without judging or reacting. If you notice any distractions, gently bring your attention back to your breath and body. You can also use a mantra, a word, or a sound, to help you focus and calm your mind. You can also use a timer, a bell, or a music, to help you keep track of the time and end your meditation.

Hold this pose for as long as you like, or for 5 to 10 minutes. Then, gently open your eyes and return to the present moment. You can also stretch your arms and legs, or massage your face and head, to awaken your senses and body.

Tips and modifications:

You can adjust the duration and difficulty of the sequence, depending on your time, energy, and ability. You can do more or less repetitions, or hold the poses for longer or shorter periods of time. You can also skip or add some poses or movements, depending on your preference and goals.

You can also use some props, such as a cushion, a blanket, a towel, a strap, a block, or a pillow, to make your practice more comfortable and effective. You can use items that you already have at home, or buy them online or at a local store.

You can also play some soothing music, light some candles, or use some aromatherapy, if you like. You can also invite a friend, a family member, or a pet to join you, if you want some company and fun.

Contraindications and precautions

This sequence is generally safe and suitable for everyone, but if you have any medical or health issues, consult your doctor or a yoga therapist before doing this sequence, or any other chair yoga practice. You can also ask them for advice on how to modify the sequence to suit your specific needs and conditions.

- If you have any lower back, hip, knee, ankle, shoulder, wrist, neck, or spinal issues, be careful not to overstretch or aggravate them. You can use props or modify the pose or the sequence to make it more comfortable and safe for you.

- If you have any high blood pressure, glaucoma, or heart issues, be careful not to lift or lower your head too much or hold your breath.

You can keep your head in line with your spine, or use props or modify the pose or the sequence to make it more gentle and safe for you
Here is a possible section on

CHAPTER 4: Chair Yoga Tips and Precautions for Sciatica Relief

In this chapter, you will find some useful tips and precautions that can help you practice chair yoga safely and effectively for sciatica relief. These tips and precautions will help you avoid common chair yoga mistakes and injuries, and enhance your chair yoga experience and results. They will also help you monitor your progress and pain levels, and know when to consult your doctor or a yoga therapist.

For each tip and precaution, you will find the following information:

- The name and description of the tip or precaution, along with an illustration
- The reason and benefit of the tip or precaution for sciatica relief
- The examples and suggestions on how to apply the tip or precaution to your chair yoga practice

Before you start, make sure you have a chair and some space around it. You can also use some props, such as a cushion, a blanket, a towel, a strap, a block, or a pillow, to make your practice more comfortable and effective. You can use items that you already have at home, or buy them online or at a local store.

Remember to breathe deeply and slowly throughout your practice, and pay attention to your body and sensations. Do not force or strain yourself, and respect your limits. If you feel any pain or discomfort, stop or modify the pose or the sequence. You can also take a break or rest whenever you need to. Listen to your body and its wisdom, and enjoy your practice.

Here are the chair yoga tips and precautions for sciatica relief:

- How to breathe properly during chair yoga

This is a tip that helps you breathe in a way that supports your chair yoga practice and sciatica relief. It helps you breathe through your nose, and use your diaphragm, abdomen, and chest, to inhale and exhale fully and smoothly. It also helps you synchronize your breath and movement, and use your breath as a guide and a tool.

Reason and benefit: Breathing properly during chair yoga can help you relieve sciatica pain and discomfort by relaxing your nervous system, and easing any tension or inflammation. It can also help you improve your circulation and oxygen flow, and nourish your muscles and nerves. It can also help you calm your mind and emotions, and enhance your focus and awareness.

Examples and suggestions: To breathe properly during chair yoga, follow these steps:

Sit on a chair with your feet flat on the floor and your knees bent at 90 degrees. You can place a cushion or a

blanket under your feet or your hips, if needed.

Lengthen your spine and lift your chest. Place your hands on your thighs or on the sides of the chair. Keep your head in line with your spine, and look straight ahead or slightly down. This is the Seated Mountain Pose. (See Chapter 1 for more details)

Close your mouth and breathe through your nose. Feel the air enter and exit your nostrils, and notice the temperature and quality of your breath. You can also use a tissue, a cotton ball, or a finger, to block one nostril at a time, and breathe through the other nostril, to balance your breath and energy. This is the Alternate Nostril Breathing. (See below for more details)

Breathe deeply and slowly, and use your diaphragm, abdomen, and chest, to inhale and exhale fully and smoothly. Feel your abdomen and chest expand and contract, and notice the rhythm and pace of your breath. You can also place your hands on your abdomen and chest, to feel the movement and feedback. This is the Three-Part Breathing. (See below for more details)

Synchronize your breath and movement, and use your breath as a guide and a tool. Inhale when you lengthen, lift, or open your body, and exhale when you bend, lower, or close your body. Use your breath to initiate and support your movement, and to deepen and relax your pose. You can also use your breath to adjust your intensity and duration, and to monitor your comfort and pain levels.

This is the Breath-Awareness Movement. (See below for more

To do the Alternate Nostril Breathing, follow these steps:

- Inhale and lengthen your spine and lift your chest. Place your right hand on your right knee or on the side of the chair, and bring your left hand to your face. Keep your head in line with your spine, and look straight ahead or slightly down. This is the Seated Mountain Pose with Left Hand to Face.

Exhale and close your left nostril with your left thumb, and breathe through your right nostril. Feel the air enter and exit your right nostril, and notice the temperature and quality of your breath. Breathe deeply and slowly, and use your diaphragm, abdomen, and chest, to inhale and exhale fully and smoothly.

- Inhale through your right nostril, and close your right nostril with your left ring finger, and open your left nostril. Breathe through your left nostril. Feel the air enter and exit your left nostril, and notice the temperature and quality of your breath. Breathe deeply and slowly, and use your diaphragm, abdomen, and chest, to inhale and exhale fully and smoothly. Exhale through your left nostril, and close your left nostril with your left thumb, and open your right nostril. Breathe through your right nostril. Feel the air enter and exit your right nostril, and notice the temperature and quality of your breath. Breathe deeply and slowly, and use your diaphragm, abdomen, and chest, to inhale and exhale fully and smoothly.

Repeat this cycle for as long as you like, or for 5 to 10 times. Then, lower your left hand, and breathe through both nostrils. This is the Seated Mountain Pose.

To do the Three-Part Breathing, follow these steps:

- Inhale and lengthen your spine and lift your chest. Place your hands on your abdomen and chest, or on your thighs or on the sides of the chair. Keep your head in line with your spine, and look straight ahead or slightly down. This is the Seated Mountain Pose with Hands on Abdomen and Chest.

- Exhale and empty your lungs completely, and draw your navel toward your spine. Feel your abdomen contract, and notice the pressure and release of your breath.

- Inhale and fill your lungs from the bottom to the top, and expand your abdomen, chest, and collarbones. Feel your abdomen and chest expand, and notice the volume and space of your breath.

Exhale and empty your lungs from the top to the bottom, and relax your collarbones, chest, and abdomen. Feel your abdomen and chest contract, and notice the pressure and release of your breath.

Repeat this cycle for as long as you like, or for 5 to 10 times. Then, breathe normally. This is the Seated Mountain Pose.

To do the Breath-Awareness Movement, follow these steps:

Inhale and lengthen your spine and lift your chest. Place your hands on your thighs or on the sides of the chair. Keep your head in line with your spine, and look straight ahead or slightly down. This is the Seated Mountain Pose.

Exhale and hinge from your hips, and fold your torso over your legs. Bring your hands to the floor, to your ankles, to your shins, or to your knees. Relax your head, neck, and shoulders. This is the Seated Forward Bend. (See Chapter 1 for more details)

Inhale and lift your torso halfway up, and place your hands on your shins or on the sides of the chair. Lengthen your spine and lift your chest. Look straight ahead or slightly down. This is the Seated Halfway Lift. (See Chapter 2 for more details)

- Exhale and fold your torso over your legs again. Bring your hands to the floor, to your ankles, to your shins, or to your knees. Relax your head, neck, and shoulders. This is the Seated Forward Bend.

- Inhale and raise your torso and arms up, and bring your palms together. Look up at your hands, or keep your head in line with your spine. This is the Seated Mountain Pose with Prayer Hands. (See Chapter 2 for more details)

- Exhale and lower your arms to shoulder level, and turn your torso to the right. Bring your left hand to the outside of your right knee, and your right hand to the back of the chair or to your right hip. Look over your right shoulder, or keep your head in line with your spine. This is the Seated Spinal Twist to the right. (See Chapter 1 for more details)

- Inhale and return to the center, and raise your arms to shoulder level. This is the Seated Mountain Pose with Arms Out. (See Chapter 2 for more details)

- Exhale and turn your torso to the left. Bring your right hand to the outside of your left knee, and your left hand to the back of the chair or to your left hip. Look over your left shoulder, or keep your head in line with your spine. This is the

Seated Spinal Twist to the left. (See Chapter 1 for more details)

Here is a possible section on "how to modify chair yoga poses to suit your needs and abilities" for a book on "Sciatica chair yoga for seniors over 60: a gentle and effective way to relieve sciatica symptoms at home":

How to modify chair yoga poses to suit your needs and abilities

This is a tip that helps you adjust the chair yoga poses to make them more comfortable and safe for you, depending on your physical condition, flexibility, strength, and pain level. It helps you use some props, such as a cushion, a blanket, a towel, a strap, a block, or a pillow, to support your body and enhance your pose. It also helps you change the angle, distance, or duration of your pose, to suit your preference and goals.

Reason and benefit:

Modifying chair yoga poses can help you relieve sciatica pain and discomfort by allowing you to practice at your own pace and level, and avoid any strain or injury. It can also help you improve your posture and alignment, and prevent or reduce the compression or irritation of the sciatic nerve. It can also help you enjoy your practice more, and feel more confident and empowered.

- Examples and suggestions: To modify chair yoga poses, follow these steps:

- Choose a chair that is stable, sturdy, and comfortable for you. You can use a chair with or without arms, depending on your preference and needs. You can also use a chair with or without a back, depending on the pose and your comfort and support. You can also use a chair that is adjustable in height, or place some books or blocks under the chair legs, to raise or lower the chair seat, depending on your flexibility and comfort.

Use some props, such as a cushion, a blanket, a towel, a strap, a block, or a pillow, to make your practice more comfortable and effective. You can use items that you already have at home, or buy them online or at a local store. You can place the props under your feet, hips, knees, back, head, or hands, to support your body and enhance your pose. You can also use the props to help you reach further, bend deeper, or twist more, depending on your flexibility and needs.

Change the angle, distance, or duration of your pose, to suit your preference and goals. You can bend your knees more or less, depending on your comfort and flexibility. You can also widen your feet and legs, or cross your legs, if you want to add some variation and intensity. You can also twist your torso slightly to the right and left, or tilt your head slightly to the right and left, if you want to add some movement and stretch. You can also hold the pose for longer or shorter periods of time, depending on your comfort and endurance.

Follow the instructions, illustrations, and tips for each pose and movement, as described in the previous chapters, and pay attention to the modifications and suggestions that are provided for each pose. You can also experiment with different props and adjustments, and find what works best for you. Pay attention to your breath, body, and sensations. Do not force or strain yourself, and respect your limits. If you feel any pain or discomfort, stop or modify the pose or the sequence. You can also take a break or rest whenever you need to.

Here is a possible section on "how to avoid common chair yoga mistakes and injuries" for a book on "Sciatica chair yoga for seniors over 60: a gentle and effective way to relieve sciatica symptoms at home":

How to avoid common chair yoga mistakes and injuries

This is a precaution that helps you prevent or reduce the risk of common chair yoga mistakes and injuries that can worsen your sciatica pain and discomfort, or cause other health problems. It helps you practice chair yoga safely and effectively, and avoid any strain or damage to your muscles, joints, nerves, or organs. It also helps you improve your posture and alignment, and enhance your chair yoga experience and results.

Reason and benefit:

Avoiding common chair yoga mistakes and injuries can help you relieve sciatica pain and discomfort by allowing you to practice without any pain or harm, and heal your body and mind. It can also help you improve your circulation and oxygen flow, and nourish your muscles and nerves. It can also help you calm your mind and emotions, and enhance your focus and awareness.

Examples and suggestions: To avoid common chair yoga mistakes and injuries, follow these steps:

Choose a chair that is stable, sturdy, and comfortable for you. You can use a chair with or without arms, depending on your preference and needs. You can also use a chair with or without a back, depending on the pose and your comfort and support. You can also use a chair that is adjustable in height, or place some books or blocks under the chair legs, to raise or lower the chair seat, depending on your flexibility and comfort. Avoid using a chair that is too soft, too hard, too high, too low, too narrow, or too wide, as it can affect your posture and alignment, and cause you to lose your balance or hurt yourself.

Use some props, such as a cushion, a blanket, a towel, a strap, a block, or a pillow, to make your practice more comfortable and effective. You can use items that you already have at home, or buy them online or at a local store. You can place the props under your feet, hips, knees, back, head, or hands, to support your body and enhance your pose. You can also use the props to help you reach further, bend deeper, or twist more, depending on your flexibility and needs. Avoid using props that are too soft, too hard, too big, too small, or too slippery, as they can affect your posture and alignment, and cause you to lose your grip or hurt yourself.

Follow the instructions, illustrations, and tips for each pose and movement, as described in the previous chapters, and pay attention to the modifications and suggestions that are provided for each pose. You can also experiment with different props and adjustments, and find what works best for you. Pay attention to your breath, body, and sensations. Do not force or strain yourself, and respect your limits. If you feel any pain or discomfort, stop or modify the pose or the sequence. You can also take a break or rest whenever you need to. Avoid doing poses or movements that are too difficult, too easy, too fast, too slow, or too long, as they can affect your posture and alignment, and cause you to lose your breath or hurt yourself.

- Avoid some common chair yoga mistakes and injuries, such as:

Holding your breath or breathing too shallowly, as it can affect your circulation and oxygen flow, and cause you to feel dizzy, nauseous, or faint. Breathe deeply and slowly through your nose, and use your diaphragm, abdomen, and chest, to inhale and exhale fully and smoothly. Synchronize your breath and movement, and use your breath as a guide and a tool. (See Chapter 4 for more details)

Slouching or hunching your back, as it can affect your posture and alignment, and cause you to compress or irritate your spine, discs, nerves, or organs. Lengthen your spine and lift your chest, and relax your shoulders and neck. Keep your head in line with your spine, and look straight ahead or slightly down. Use some props or modify the pose, to support your back and head. (See Chapter 4 for more details)

Locking or hyperextending your joints, as it can affect your posture and alignment, and cause you to strain or injure your muscles, tendons, ligaments, or cartilage. Keep a slight bend in your elbows, knees, and ankles, and avoid pushing or pulling too hard. Use some props or modify the pose, to support your joints and limbs. (See Chapter 4 for more details)

Overstretching or overtwisting your muscles, as it can affect your posture and alignment, and cause you to tear or damage your muscles, fascia, or nerves. Keep a gentle and comfortable stretch in your muscles, and avoid going beyond your edge. Use some props or modify the pose, to adjust the intensity and duration of your stretch. (See Chapter 4 for more details)

Here is a possible section on "how to monitor your progress and pain level" for a book on "Sciatica chair yoga for seniors over 60: a gentle and effective way to relieve sciatica symptoms at home":

How to monitor your progress and pain level

This is a tip that helps you track your improvement and recovery from sciatica, and adjust your chair yoga practice accordingly. It helps you use some tools, such as a journal, a scale, a timer, or a tracker, to record and measure your progress and pain level. It also helps you use some indicators, such as your range of motion, your flexibility, your strength, your endurance, your sleep quality, your mood, and your satisfaction, to evaluate your progress and pain level.

Reason and benefit

Monitoring your progress and pain level can help you relieve sciatica pain and discomfort by allowing you to see your achievements and challenges, and celebrate your successes and learn from your mistakes. It can also help you customize your chair yoga practice to suit your needs and goals, and avoid any overexertion or underestimation. It can also help you motivate yourself and stay committed to your chair yoga practice, and enjoy your journey and results.

Examples and suggestions: To monitor your progress and pain level, follow these steps:

Choose some tools, such as a journal, a scale, a timer, or a tracker, to record and measure your progress and pain level. You can use items that you already have at home, or buy them online or at a local store. You can also use some apps or websites, such as [MySciatica], [Sciatica Tracker], or [PainScale], to help you monitor your progress and pain level. (See below for more details)

Choose some indicators, such as your range of motion, your flexibility, your strength, your endurance, your sleep quality, your mood, and your satisfaction, to evaluate your progress and pain level. You can use some tests, such as the [Straight Leg Raise Test], the [Sit and Reach Test], the [Chair Stand Test], the [Six-Minute Walk Test], the [Pittsburgh Sleep Quality Index], the [Positive and Negative Affect Schedule], or the [Patient Satisfaction Questionnaire], to help you assess your indicators. (See below for more details)

Record and measure your progress and pain level before, during, and after your chair yoga practice, or at regular intervals, such as daily, weekly, or monthly. Use your tools and indicators to collect and analyze your data, and compare your results over time. You can also use some charts, graphs, or tables, to visualize and summarize your data, and make it easier to understand and interpret. You can also use some statistics, such as the mean, median, mode, standard deviation, or correlation, to calculate and describe your data, and make it more accurate and reliable.

Evaluate your progress and pain level, and adjust your chair yoga practice accordingly. Use your data and results to identify your strengths and weaknesses, and celebrate your achievements and challenges. You can also use your data and results to customize your chair yoga practice to suit your needs and goals, and avoid any overexertion or underestimation. You can also use your data and results to motivate yourself and stay committed to your chair yoga practice, and enjoy your journey and results.

To use the tools, such as the apps or websites, to monitor your progress and pain level, follow these steps: Download the app or visit the website, and create an account or log in. You can use [MySciatica], [Sciatica Tracker], or [PainScale], or any other app or website that you prefer or trust. These are some examples of apps or websites that are designed to help you monitor your progress and pain level for sciatica.

Follow the instructions and prompts, and enter your personal information, such as your name, age, gender, height, weight, medical history, and current condition. You can also enter your chair yoga information, such as your frequency, duration, intensity, and type of chair yoga practice. You can also enter your goals and expectations, such as your desired pain level, range of motion, flexibility, strength, endurance, sleep quality, mood, and satisfaction

Use the app or website to record and measure your progress and pain level before, during, and after your chair yoga practice, or at regular intervals, such as daily, weekly, or monthly.

You can use the app or website to enter your data and results, such as your pain level, range of motion, flexibility, strength, endurance, sleep quality, mood, and satisfaction. You can also use the app or website to take some tests, such as the Straight Leg Raise Test, the Sit and Reach Test, the Chair Stand Test, the Six-Minute Walk Test, the Pittsburgh Sleep Quality Index, the Positive and Negative Affect Schedule, or the Patient Satisfaction Questionnaire, to help you assess your indicators. You can also use the app or website to take some photos, videos, or audios, to help you document your progress and pain level.

Use the app or website to analyze and compare your data and results over time. You can use the app or website to view your charts, graphs, or tables, that visualize and summarize your data and results, and make it easier to understand and interpret. You can also use the app or website to view your statistics, that calculate and describe your data and results, and make it more accurate and reliable. You can also use the app or website to view your feedback, that provide you with some tips, suggestions, or recommendations, based on your data and results, and help you improve your chair yoga practice and sciatica relief.

To use the tests, such as the Straight Leg Raise Test, the Sit and Reach Test, the Chair Stand Test, the Six-Minute Walk Test, the Pittsburgh Sleep Quality Index, the Positive and Negative Affect Schedule, or the Patient Satisfaction Questionnaire, to assess your indicators, follow these steps:

Choose a test that corresponds to your indicator, such as the Straight Leg Raise Test for your range of motion, the Sit and Reach Test for your flexibility, the Chair Stand Test for your strength, the Six-Minute Walk Test for your endurance, the Pittsburgh Sleep Quality Index for your sleep quality, the Positive and

Negative Affect Schedule for your mood, or the Patient Satisfaction Questionnaire for your satisfaction. You can use these tests, or any other tests that you prefer or trust. These are some examples of tests that are designed to help you assess your indicators for sciatica relief.

Follow the instructions and procedures, and perform the test correctly and safely. You can use some tools, such as a ruler, a tape measure, a stopwatch, or a scale, to help you perform the test, if needed. You can also use some props, such as a cushion, a blanket, a towel, a strap, a block, or a pillow, to make the test more comfortable and effective, if needed. You can also ask a friend, a family member, or a helper, to assist you with the test, if needed.

Record and measure your data and results, and compare them over time. You can use some tools, such as a journal, a scale, a timer, or a tracker, to record and measure your data and results, if needed. You can also use some charts, graphs, or tables, to visualize and summarize your data and results, and make it easier to understand and interpret, if needed. You can also use some statistics, such as the mean, median, mode, standard deviation, or correlation, to calculate and describe your data and results, and make it more accurate and reliable, if needed.

Here is a possible section on "when to consult your doctor or a yoga therapist" for a book on "Sciatica chair yoga for seniors over 60: a gentle and effective way to relieve sciatica symptoms at home":

When to consult your doctor or a yoga therapist

This is a precaution that helps you know when to seek professional help and advice for your sciatica condition and chair yoga practice. It helps you recognize the signs and symptoms that indicate a serious or worsening problem, and avoid any further complications or damage. It also helps you find a qualified and experienced doctor or yoga therapist, who can diagnose and treat your sciatica condition, and guide and support your chair yoga practice.

Reason and benefit

Consulting your doctor or a yoga therapist can help you relieve sciatica pain and discomfort by allowing you to get a proper diagnosis and treatment, and avoid any misdiagnosis or mistreatment. It can also help you improve your chair yoga practice and sciatica relief, by providing you with some personalized and professional tips, suggestions, or recommendations, based on your medical history, current condition, and specific needs and goals.

Examples and suggestions: To consult your doctor or a yoga therapist, follow these steps:

Consult your doctor or a yoga therapist before starting or changing your chair yoga practice, or any other physical activity, especially if you have any medical or health issues, such as lower back, hip, knee, ankle, shoulder, wrist, neck, or spinal issues, high blood pressure, glaucoma, or heart issues. You can also consult your doctor or a yoga therapist if you are pregnant, breastfeeding, or menstruating, as some chair yoga poses or movements may not be suitable or safe for you. You can also consult your doctor or a yoga

therapist if you are taking any medication, supplements, or herbs, as some chair yoga poses or movements may interact or interfere with them.

Consult your doctor or a yoga therapist if you experience any of the following signs and symptoms, as they may indicate a serious or worsening problem, and require immediate medical attention or intervention:

Severe, sharp, or shooting pain in your lower back, buttocks, or legs, that does not improve or worsens with rest, movement, or medication.

Numbness, tingling, or weakness in your lower back, buttocks, or legs, that affects your mobility, balance, or coordination.

Loss of bladder or bowel control, or sexual function, due to nerve compression or damage.
- Fever, chills, sweats, or infection, due to inflammation or infection of the spine, discs, nerves, or organs.

Trauma, injury, or fracture, due to a fall, accident, or impact, that affects your spine, discs, nerves, or organs

Consult your doctor or a yoga therapist if you have any questions, doubts, or concerns about your sciatica condition or chair yoga practice, or if you want to learn more or get some advice. You can also consult your doctor or a yoga therapist if you want to monitor your progress and pain level, or if you want to modify or customize your chair yoga practice to suit your needs and goals.

Find a qualified and experienced doctor or yoga therapist, who can diagnose and treat your sciatica condition, and guide and support your chair yoga practice. You can ask your family, friends, or colleagues for some referrals or recommendations, or you can search online or in your local area for some reviews or ratings.

You can also check the credentials, qualifications, and certifications of the doctor or yoga therapist, and make sure they are licensed, registered, and insured. You can also contact the doctor or yoga therapist, and ask them some questions, such as their background, experience, approach, methods, fees, and availability. You can also schedule an appointment or a consultation with the doctor or yoga therapist, and meet them in person or online, and see if you feel comfortable and confident with them.